Dx/Rx:
Human Papilloma Virus

Don S. Dizon, MD
Associate Professor
The Warren Alpert Medical School of Brown University
Director of Medical Oncology and Integrative Care
Co-Director, The Center for Sexuality, Intimacy, and Fertility
Women and Infants Hospital
Providence, Rhode Island

Ashley R. Stuckey, MD
Assistant Professor of Obstetrics and Gynecology
The Warren Alpert Medical School of Brown University
Program in Women's Oncology
Women and Infants Hospital
Brown University School of Medicine
Providence, Rhode Island

Michael L. Krychman, MD
Executive Director
Southern California Center for Sexual Health and
    Survivorship Medicine
Associate Clinical Professor
University of Southern California
Associate Clinical Professor
University of California Irvine
Newport Beach, California

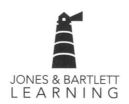

JONES & BARTLETT
L E A R N I N G

World Headquarters

Jones & Bartlett Learning
40 Tall Pine Drive
Sudbury, MA 01776
978-443-5000
info@jblearning.com
www.jblearning.com

Jones & Bartlett Learning Canada
6339 Ormindale Way
Mississauga, Ontario L5V 1J2
Canada

Jones & Bartlett Learning International
Barb House, Barb Mews
London W6 7PA
United Kingdom

Jones & Bartlett Learning books and products are available through most bookstores and online booksellers. To contact Jones & Bartlett Learning directly, call 800-832-0034, fax 978-443-8000, or visit our website, www.jblearning.com.

Substantial discounts on bulk quantities of Jones & Bartlett Learning publications are available to corporations, professional associations, and other qualified organizations. For details and specific discount information, contact the special sales department at Jones & Bartlett Learning via the above contact information or send an email to specialsales@jblearning.com.

The authors, editor, and publisher have made every effort to provide accurate information. However, they are not responsible for errors, omissions, or for any outcomes related to the use of the contents of this book and take no responsibility for the use of the products and procedures described. Treatments and side effects described in this book may not be applicable to all people; likewise, some people may require a dose or experience a side effect that is not described herein. Drugs and medical devices are discussed that may have limited availability controlled by the Food and Drug Administration (FDA) for use only in a research study or clinical trial. Research, clinical practice, and government regulations often change the accepted standard in this field. When consideration is being given to use of any drug in the clinical setting, the healthcare provider or reader is responsible for determining FDA status of the drug, reading the package insert, and reviewing prescribing information for the most up-to-date recommendations on dose, precautions, and contraindications, and determining the appropriate usage for the product. This is especially important in the case of drugs that are new or seldom used.

Production Credits

Executive Publisher: Christopher Davis
Editorial Assistant: Sara Cameron
Associate Production Editor: Jill Morton
Associate Marketing Manager: Katie Hennessy
V.P., Manufacturing and Inventory
  Control: Therese Connell
Project Management: Thistle Hill Publishing
  Services, LLC

Composition: Dedicated Business Solutions
Cover Design: Kate Ternullo
Cover Image: © Michael Taylor/
  ShutterStock, Inc.
Printing and Binding: Malloy Incorporated
Cover Printing: Malloy Incorporated

Library of Congress Cataloging-in-Publication Data
Dizon, Don S.
  Dx/Rx. Human papilloma virus / Don S. Dizon, Ashley R. Stuckey, Michael L. Krychman.
    p. ; cm.
  Other title: Human papilloma virus
  Includes bibliographical references and index.
  ISBN-13: 978-0-7637-8161-3 (pbk.)
  ISBN-10: 0-7637-8161-4 (pbk.)
  1. Papillomavirus diseases. I. Stuckey, Ashley R. II. Krychman, Michael L. III. Title.
IV. Title: Human papilloma virus.
  [DNLM: 1. Papillomavirus Infections. 2. Alphapapillomavirus. 3. Papillomavirus
Vaccines. QZ 200]
  RC168.P15D58 2011
  616.9'11—dc22
                                    2010033531
6048

Printed in the United States of America
14 13 12 11 10   10 9 8 7 6 5 4 3 2 1

CHAPTER 1

Epidemiology and Risk Factors

■ Background

- Zur Hausen in the 1970s proposed that the human papilloma virus (HPV) played a role in the development of genital tract neoplasia.

- HPV sequences were then discovered in the 1980s in genital warts.

- The direct medical costs associated with the prevention and treatment of HPV-related anogenital warts and cervical disease in the United States are estimated to be $4.0 billion annually.

- In a study by Pirotta et al., 331 women recruited from the outpatient clinics of a major tertiary hospital in Melbourne, Australia, were surveyed on the psychosocial impact following an HPV-related diagnosis.[1] Women diagnosed with an HPV-related condition were more likely to be informed about HPV, compared with women who had normal Pap smears. Still, being informed did not translate into a lesser degree of worry or concern. In fact, they found that women diagnosed with CIN 2-3, or external genital warts, had a significant psychosocial impact following diagnosis than those with normal Pap smears.

- Productivity losses due to deaths from cervical cancer are estimated to be $1.3 billion annually.[2,3]

- External genital warts also represent a significant economic burden with associated quality-adjusted life year (QALY) loss, ranging from 0.0045 (95% CI: 0.0014–0.0078) to 0.023 (95% CI: 0.0072–0.039).[4]

■ HPV Incidence and Prevalence (Table 1.1)

- HPV is the most common genital infection in the United States, and men and women are at equal risk of infection. The lifetime risk of at least one HPV infection in women is 75%.[5,6]
- The World Health Organization estimates the prevalence of HPV infection to be 440 million people infected worldwide.
- HPV is more common in younger age groups, especially young women in their teens and early 20s.
  - In a nationally representative study of women in the United States, 25% of people between ages 14 and 19 years and 45% of people between ages 20 and 24 years were HPV positive.[7]
  - HPV is often acquired during the initial few months of first sexual intercourse. Approximately 30% of university women become HPV positive within 1 year of first intercourse and more than 50% of college-age women acquire HPV infection within 3 years of first intercourse.[8]
- For high-risk HPV types, there is a bimodal distribution of infection that is seen most commonly in women younger than 20 years of age and then again in women around 50 years of age. Infection with the low-risk types of HPV decreases with age.[9]
- Healthcare professionals believe it is important to educate patients about viral transmission and HPV-associated diseases. The psychosocial ramifications, however, cannot be ignored; patients should be reassured about the high prevalence (at least 75% of men and women will be infected in their lifetime) of the virus, that most immune systems will clear the virus, and that often no treatment is warranted.

■ Risk Factors for HPV Infection

- Early onset of sexual activity
- Multiple sexual partners
- History of sexually transmitted infections

Table 1.1   Worldwide Data for Cancers Attributable to Infection with Oncogenic HPV

Site	Total Number of Cancers	Attributable Fraction (%)	Attributable Cancers	% of All Cancer
Cervix	492,800	10	492,800	4.5
Penis	26,300	40	10,500	0.1
Vulva, Vagina	40,000	40	16,000	0.2
Anus	30,400	90	27,400	0.2
Mouth	274,100	3	8200	0.1
Oropharynx	52,100	12	6300	0.1
All sites	10,843,600		561,200	5.2

Source: Adapted from Parkin DM. The global health burden of infection-associated cancers in the year 2002. *Int J Cancer.* 2006;118:3030–3044.

- Early age at first pregnancy
- Tobacco use
  - Smoking favors HPV persistence and subsequent neoplastic development[10,11]

■ HPV Transmission

- HPV can be transmitted by vaginal, anal, or oral intercourse. Condoms are only partially protective against transmission. Microtrauma increases the risk of infection of the cervical epithelium.[12,13]
- Vertical transmission of HPV from mother to infant is uncommon.[14,15]
- HPV is an intraepithelial microbe and grows in the basal epithelial cells of the cervix. HPV is typically cleared by a healthy immune system in 12–18 months, but the proportion of women with persistent infection ranges from 1% to 20%.
- For women, HPV is the single most important biologic risk factor for developing genital warts as well as both precancerous lesions and invasive cancers of the genital track (cervix, vulva, vagina, and anal canal). In men, HPV is an important risk for the development of both anal and penile cancers.
- Following HPV infection, detectable HPV antibodies are seen in only 50% of women and in low levels.
  - Low antibody levels may not provide protection against future HPV infection.[16,17]
  - Antibodies to HPV have not been shown to protect against ongoing infection.[18]

■ References

1. Pirotta M, Ung L, Stein A, et al. The psychosocial burden of human papillomavirus related disease and screening interventions. *Sex Transm Infect.* 2009;85:508–513.
2. Insinga RP, Dasbach EJ, Elbasha EH. Assessing the annual economic burden of preventing and treating anogenital human papillomavirus-related disease in the US: analytic framework and review of the literature. *Pharmacoeconomics.* 2005;23:1107–1122.

3. Insinga RP. Annual productivity costs due to cervical cancer mortality in the United States. *Womens Health Issues.* 2006;16:236–242.

4. Woodhall SC, Jit M, Cai C, et al. Cost of treatment and QALYs lost due to genital warts: data for the economic evaluation of HPV vaccines in the United Kingdom. *Sex Transm Dis.* 2009;36:515–521.

5. Cates W. Estimates of the incidence and prevalence of sexually transmitted diseases in the United States. American Social Health Association Panel. *Sex Transm Dis.* 1999;26(4)(suppl):S2–S7.

6. Baseman JG, Koutsky LA. The epidemiology of human papillomavirus infections. *J Clin Virol.* 2005;32(suppl 1): S16–S24.

7. Dunne EF, Unger ER, Sternberg M, et al. Prevalence of HPV infection among females in the United States. *JAMA.* 2007;297:813–819.

8. Winer RL, Feng Q, Hughes JP, et al. Risk of female human papillomavirus acquisition associated with first male sex partner. *J Infect Dis.* 2008;197:279–282.

9. Munoz N, Mendez F, Posso H, et al. Incidence, duration, and determinants of cervical human papillomavirus infection in a cohort of Colombian women with normal cytological results. *J Infect Dis.* 2004;190:2077–2087.

10. McIntyre-Seltman K, Castle PE, Guido R, et al; ALTS Group. Smoking is a risk factor for cervical intraepithelial neoplasia grade 3 among oncogenic human papillomavirus DNA-positive women with equivocal or mildly abnormal cytology. *Cancer Epidemiol Biomarkers Prev.* 2005;14:1165–1170.

11. Tsai HT, Tsai YM, Yang SF, et al. Lifetime cigarette smoke and second-hand smoke and cervical intraepithelial neoplasm—a community-based case-control study. *Gynecol Oncol.* 2007;105:181–188.

12. Stanley M, Lowy DR, Frazer I. Prophylactic HPV vaccines: underlying mechanisms. *Vaccine.* 2006;24(suppl 3): S106–S113.

13. Tindle RW. Immune evasion in human papillomavirus-associated cancers. *Nat Rev Cancer.* 2002;2(1):59–65.

14. Saslow D, Castle PE, Cox JT, et al. American Cancer Society Guideline for HPV vaccine use to prevent cervical cancer and its precursors. *CA Cancer J Clin.* 2007;57(1):7–28.

15. Bosch FX, Qiao Y-L, Castellsague X. The epidemiology of human papillomavirus infection and its association with cervical cancer. *Int J Gynaecol Obstet.* 2006;94(suppl 1): S8–S21.

16. Stanley M. Immune responses to human papillomavirus. *Vaccine*. 2006;24(suppl 1):S16–S22.

17. Viscidi RP, Schiffman M, Hildesheim A, et al. Seroreactivity to human papillomavirus (HPV) types 16, 18, or 31 and risk of subsequent HPV infection: results from a population-based study in Costa Rica. *Cancer Epidemiol Biomarkers Prev*. 2004;13(2):324–327.

18. Hildesheim A, Herrero R, Wacholder S, et al; Costa Rican HPV Vaccine Trial Group. Effect of human papillomavirus 16/18 L1 virus-like particle vaccine among young women with preexisting infection: a randomized trial. *JAMA*. 2007; 15;298(7):743–753.

CHAPTER 2

The HPV Genome

■ HPV Subtypes

- ■ HPV subtypes are classified based on their high- or low-risk oncogenic behavior (**Table 2.1**[1]).
- ■ There are more than 100 genetic subtypes of the HPV virus (**Table 2.2**).[2,3]
  - • Forty are known to infect the anogenital region.
  - • Fifteen are considered to be oncogenic.
  - • HPV 16 and HPV 18 are associated with the highest risk, causing about 50% and 20% of all cervical cancers, respectively.[4]

■ HPV Genome

- ■ Viral characteristics
  - • The human papilloma virus is a small, nonenveloped icosahedral double-stranded circular DNA virus that infects mucosal epithelial or cutaneous surfaces.
  - • HPV is an intraepithelial pathogen than has no blood-borne phase. It does not lyse the keratinocytes and is almost invisible to the host. It encodes proteins that inhibit apoptosis and downregulates the interferon response.
  - • Its 8-kb circular genome encodes seven early proteins (E1–E7) and two late nucleocapsid proteins (L1–L2) (**Figure 2.1**).
    - ■ The early genes are responsible for viral DNA replication (E1, E2), RNA transcription (E2), cytoskeleton reorganization (E4), and cell transformation (E5, E6, E7).[5,6]
    - ■ The late genes encode the viral capsid components and other nonstructural proteins.

Table 2.1 HPV Subtypes

High-Risk Types: 16, 18, 31, 33, 35, 39, 45, 51, 52, 56, 58, 59, 68, 73, 82

Low-Risk Types: 6, 11, 40, 42, 43, 44, 54, 61, 70, 72, 81, CP6108

Potentially High-Risk Types: 26, 53, 66

Source: Adapted from Robison K, Dizon DS. *Dx/Rx: Cervical Cancer. Diagnosis and Treatment of Pre-cancerous Lesions (CIN) and Cervical Cancer.* 2nd ed. Sudbury, MA: Jones & Bartlett Learning; 2011:3.

Table 2.2 HPV Types Associated with Common Human Diseases

Human-Disease	HPV-type
Warts	
Common Warts (verrucae vulgaris)	1,2,4,26,2,29,41,57,65
Plantar Warts	1,2,4,63
Flat Warts (face)	3,10,27,28,38,41,49
Anogenital Warts	6,11,30,42,43,44,45,51,52,54
Respiratory Papillomatosis	6,11
Cervical Dysplasia	6,11,16,18,30,31,33,34,35,39, 40,42,43,44,45,51,52,53,56, 57,58,59,61,62,64,66,67,68,69
Cervical Cancer	16, 18
Penile Cancer	16, 18
Vulvar Cancer	6, 11, 16, 18
Vaginal Cancer	16
Anal Cancer	16, 31, 32, 33
Oral cancer	16, 18
Epidermodysplasia Verruciformis	
Benign	2,3,10,12,15,19,36,47,50
Malignant	5,8,9,10,14,17,20,21,22,23,24 25,37,38

Source: Adapted from Dizon DS, Krychman MA. *Questions & Answers About HPV.* Sudbury, MA: Jones & Bartlett Learning; 2011.

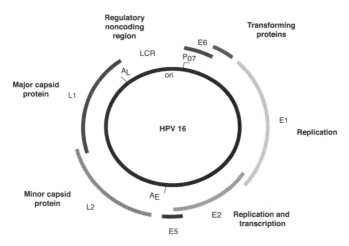

Figure 2.1 The human papilloma virus (HPV) genome.
Source: Adapted from Robison K, Dizon DS. *Dx/Rx: Cervical Cancer. Diagnosis and Treatment of Pre-cancerous Lesions (CIN) and Cervical Cancer.* 2nd ed. Sudbury, MA: Jones & Bartlett Learning; 2011:4.

- E2 regulates the expression of all other viral genes and is involved in the repression of E6 and E7.
- Mechanism of infection
  - HPV infection occurs only in keratinocytes undergoing differentiation.
  - The epithelial basement membrane has been identified as the primary site of virus binding during genital tract infection in vivo.[7]
  - Virions bind initially to the basement membrane before transfer to the basal keratinocyte cell surface.
  - Capsids are transferred to a second receptor present on the cell surface. Interaction with the second receptor induces conformational changes triggering endocytosis.
  - L1 and L2 are capsid proteins necessary for infection.
    - L1 likely provides the binding site for the uptake receptor.
    - L2, a minor capsid protein, allows escape of the viral genome from the endosome.[8]
  - The viral genome is integrated into host cell chromosomes, and the virus parasitizes the stem cells, where the E1 and E2 proteins initiate replication.[9]

- The HPV infective cycle is a multistep process and may be susceptible to neutralizing antibodies for several hours.
- Mechanism of neoplastic transformation
  - E2 is disrupted when HPV is integrated into the host DNA. E2 is a transcriptional repressor of E6 and E7, and disruption of E2 results in upregulation of E6 and E7. This elevated expression of E6 and E7 causes disruption of the cell cycle regulation and genomic instability contributing to HPV-associated cancers.[6]
- HPV is intimately involved with tumor suppressors.[10]
  - The E6 and E7 proteins afford the oncogenic potential to HPV.
  - E6 binds p53, causing ubiquitination and degradation of the tumor suppressor.
  - E7 binds and inhibits pRb, another tumor suppressor.
- HPV is the causative agent in both benign and malignant lesions.[11,12]
  - In benign lesions, the HPV genome exists in episomal form, allowing normal transcription and translation of the E2 gene, which suppresses the products of the E6 and E7 genes.
  - In malignant lesions, the HPV genome incorporates itself into the host cell, interrupting the E2 reading frame, thereby disrupting the suppression of E6 and E7.
- p16 expression may correlate with the presence of HPV.[13]
  - p16 is positive in 35–50% CIN 1 and in 70–100% CIN 2-3.
  - p16 has better correlation with high-risk HPV; therefore, histological indetermination of a CIN lesion is more likely HPV negative or of low-risk type if p16 is negative.

■ Natural History of HPV

- HPV infection occurs most often without malignant transformation with the viral DNA isolated from host DNA in an episome. In contrast, the viral DNA integrates into host DNA during malignant transformation.

- Rate of clearance of HPV infection over 5 years is approximately 90%.[11,14]
- Most HPV infections resolve within 1–2 years.[15,16]
  - First, the cell-mediated response occurs, which results in clearance of warts and low-grade lesions.
  - At 6–12 months, anti-L1 antibody leads to seroconversion. Approximately 50% of females seroconvert in 18 months.
  - At 8–14 months, 90% of people's immune system clears the virus.
- There are two types of antibodies to HPV: neutralizing and nonneutralizing antibodies. Successful host immune response includes both humoral and cell-mediated immune responses.[9,10,12,17–19]
- There are different mechanisms by which HPV infections can become persistent by evading the immune system.
  - HPV infects and multiplies in keratinocytes, which have a short life span. HPV therefore does not destroy the host cell or trigger apoptosis-induced inflammation or immune response.[20,21]
  - HPV causes downregulation of interferon genes that have antiviral and antiproliferative properties.[22,23]
  - Carcinogenesis is associated with the expression of proteins E6 and E7, which inactivate tumor suppressors p53 and retinoblastoma protein.[24]

■ References

1. Robison K, Dizon DS. *Dx/Rx: Cervical Cancer. Diagnosis and Treatment of Pre-cancerous Lesions (CIN) and Cervical Cancer.* 2nd ed. Sudbury, MA: Jones & Bartlett Learning; 2011:4.
2. Munoz N, Bosch FX, deSanjose S, et al. Epidemiologic classification of human papillomavirus types associated with cervical cancer. *New Engl J Med.* 2003;348:518–527.
3. Schiffman M, Herrero R, DeSalle R, et al. The carcinogenicity of human papillomavirus types reflects viral evolution. *Virology.* 2005;337:76–84.
4. Munoz N, Bosch FX, Castellsagué X, et al. Against which human papillomavirus types shall we vaccinate and screen? The international perspective. *Int J Cancer.* 2004;111:278–285.

5. Dizon DS, Krychman MJ. *Questions & Answers About Human Papilloma Virus (HPV)*. Sudbury, MA: Jones & Bartlett Learning; 2011.

6. Monie A, Hung C, Roden R, et al. Cervarix™: a vaccine for the prevention of HPV 16,18-associated cervical cancer. *Biologics*. 2008;2(1):107–113.

7. Roberts JN, Buck CB, Thompson CD, et al. Genital transmission of HPV in a mouse model is potentiated by nonoxynol-9 and inhibited by carrageenan. *Nat Med*. 2007;13(7):857–861.

8. Kämper N, Day PM, Nowak T, et al. A membrane-destabilizing peptide in capsid protein L2 is required for egress of papillomavirus genomes from endosomes. *J Virol*. 2006;80(2):759–768.

9. Sherman ME, Schiffman MH, Strickler H, et al. Prospects for a prophylactic HPV vaccine: rationale and future implications for cervical cancer screening. *Diagn Cytopathol*. 1998;18(1):5–9.

10. Zur Hausen H. Papillomaviruses and cancer: from basic studies to clinical application. *Nat Rev Cancer*. 2002;2:342–350.

11. Elfgren K, Kalantari M, Moberger B, et al. A population-based five-year follow-up study of cervical human papillomavirus infection. *Am J Obstet Gynecol*. 2000;183:561–567.

12. Lowy DR, Schiller JT. Prophylactic human papillomavirus vaccines. *J Clin Invest*. 2006;116:1167–1173.

13. Eifel P, Gershenson D, Kavanaugh J, Silva E, eds. *Gynecologic Cancer*. New York, NY: Springer Science; 2006:33.

14. Khan MJ, Castle PE, Lorincz AT, et al. The elevated 10-year risk of cervical precancer and cancer in women with human papillomavirus (HPV) 16 or 18 and the possible utility of type-specific HPV testing in clinical practice. *J Natl Cancer Inst*. 2005;97:1072–1079.

15. Saslow D, Castle PE, Cox JT, et al. American Cancer Society Guideline for human papillomavirus (HPV) vaccine use to prevent cervical cancer and its precursors. *CA Cancer J Clin*. 2007;57(1):7–28.

16. Wright TC. Pathology of HPV infection at the cytologic and histologic levels: basis for a 2-tiered morphologic classification system. *Int J Gynaecol Obstet*. 2006;94(suppl 1):S22–S31.

17. Schiffman M, Castle PE. Human papillomavirus: epidemiology and public health. *Arch Pathol Lab Med*. 2003;127:930–934.

18. Ho GYF, Studentsov YY, Bierman R, et al. Natural history of human papillomavirus type 16 virus-like particle antibodies

in young women. *Cancer Epidemiol Biomarkers Prev*. 2004; 13:110–116.

19. Kast WM, Feltkamp MCW, Ressing ME, et al. Cellular immunity against human papillomavirus associated cervical cancer. *Semin Virol*. 1996;7:117–123.

20. Stanley M. Immune responses to human papillomavirus. *Vaccine*. 2006;24(suppl 1):S16–S22.

21. Stanley M, Lowy DR, Frazer I. Chapter 12: Prophylactic HPV vaccines: underlying mechanisms. *Vaccine*. 2006;24(suppl 3):S106–S113.

22. Chang YE, Laimins LA. Microarray analysis identifies interferon-inducible genes and Stat-1 as major transcriptional targets of human papillomavirus type 31. *J Virol*. 2000; 74(9):4174–4182.

23. Nees M, Geoghegan JM, Hyman T, et al. Papillomavirus type 16 oncogenes downregulate expression of interferon-responsive genes and upregulate proliferation-associated and NF-kappaB-responsive genes in cervical keratinocytes. *J Virol*. 2001;75(9):4283–4296.

24. Boulet G, Horvath C, Vanden Broeck D, et al. Human papillomavirus: E6 and E7 oncogenes. *Int J Biochem Cell Biol*. 2007;39:2006–2011.

CHAPTER 3

HPV and HIV

- HIV infection is associated with more virulent HPV-associated illness, and worsening immunosuppression increases risk of HPV-associated cancers.[1]
  - Chatuverdi et al. found that low CD4 count was associated with increased invasive anal cancer among men and a trend toward increased VIN, VAIN, and invasive cervical cancer in women.
- HIV infection and HPV illness in men:
  - Anal cancer has become one of the most common non-AIDS-defining tumors in HIV-infected individuals.
    - Anal cytology has been recommended as the primary screening tool in the at-risk population. Individuals with abnormal cytology should undergo anoscopy.[2]
  - Penile and oral HPV-associated diseases seem to be more frequent in HIV-positive men.
    - Circumcision is associated with a 35% reduction in the incidence of penile HPV.[3]
- HIV infection and HPV illness in women:
  - HPV infection is more likely to persist in HIV-positive individuals, resulting in increased risk of cervical dysplasia and invasive cancer.[4]
  - In one study of women initiating antiretroviral therapy for HIV, high-risk HPV prevalence was 78.9%, and 78.4% had multiple genotypes.[5]
  - Among women with abnormal Pap smears, the most prevalent high-risk HPV types were 16, 18, 45, 51, 53, 58, 61, 66, and 70.[5]
  - HIV-positive women, especially those with severe immunosuppression, are five times more likely than

HIV-negative women to have lower genital tract neo-plasias.[6,7]

- High HPV load in HIV-positive women with severe immunosuppression is associated with a 10-fold increase risk of CIN.[8]

- Highly active antiretroviral therapy (HAART) does not seem to impact the increased rate or persistence of HPV infections in this HIV-positive population.[9]

- HIV-positive women should be screened with Pap smears twice in the first year of diagnosis and then annually thereafter.[10]

■ References

1. Chaturvedi AK, Madeleine MM, Biggar RJ, et al. Risk of human papillomavirus-associated cancers among persons with AIDS. *J Natl Cancer Inst.* 2009;101(16):1120–1130.

2. Nahas CS, da Silva Filho EV, Sequrado AA. Screening anal dysplasia and HIV-infected patients: is there an agreement between anal Pap smear and high-resolution anoscopy-guided biopsy? *Dis Colon Rectum.* 2009;52(11);1854–1860.

3. Tobian AA, Serwadda D, Quinn TC, et al. Male circumcision for the prevention of HSV-2 and HPV infections and syphilis. *N Engl J Med.* 2009;360(13):1298–1309.

4. McKenzie ND, Kobetz EN, Hnatyszyn J, et al. Women with HIV are more commonly infected with non-16 and -18 high-risk HPV types. *Gynecol Oncol.* 2010;116(3):572–577.

5. Moodley JR, Constant D, Hoffman M, et al. Human papillomavirus prevalence, viral load and pre-cancerous lesions of the cervix in women initiating highly active antiretroviral therapy in South Africa: a cross-sectional study. *BMC Cancer.* 2009;9:275.

6. Sun XW, Ellerbrock TV, Lungu O, et al. Human papillomavirus infection in human immunodeficiency virus-seropositive women. *Obstet Gynecol.* 1995;85:680–686.

7. Harris TG, Burk RD, Palesky JM, et al. Incidence of cervical intraepithelial lesions associated with HIV serostatus, CD4 cell counts and human papillomavirus test results. *JAMA.* 2005;293:1471–1476.

8. Vermund SH, Kelley KF, Klein RS, et al. High risk of human papillomavirus infection and cervical squamous intraepithelial lesions among woman with symptomatic human immunodeficiency virus infection. *Am J Obstet Gynecol.* 1991;65:392–400.

9.   de Sanjose S, Palefsky J. Cervical and anal HIV in-
     fections in HIV positive women and men. *Virus Res.*
     2002;89(2):201–211.
10. Sexually transmitted diseases treatment guidelines, 2006.
     Centers for Disease Control and Prevention. *MMWR
     Recomm Rep.* 2006;55(RR-11):1–94. http://www.cdc.gov/
     STD/Treatment/2006/rr5511.pdf. Accessed May 8, 2010.

CHAPTER 4

HPV and Diseases of the Cervix

■ Epidemiology

- Cervical cancer is the second most common cancer in women worldwide, and in developing countries, it is the second most common cancer diagnosis and the most common cancer-related death in women.[1]
  - In 2007, there were 555,094 new cases of cervical cancer worldwide.
  - In 2007, there were 309,808 estimated deaths worldwide due to cervical cancer.
  - In the United States in 2009, there were 11,270 new cases of cervical cancer and 4,070 deaths.[2]
- Worldwide, the highest incidence rates are noted in sub-Saharan Africa, Central and South America, the Caribbean, and Southern Asia. Rates are lowest in the Middle East, most of China, and Australia.[1]
- Racial demographics:
  - Hispanic women have the highest incidence rates, followed by African American women, Caucasian, Asian, and Pacific Islander. Non-Hispanic white women have the lowest incidence rates.[3]
  - Diagnosis at an early stage is more common in white women (52%) than in African American women (44%) and in women younger than 50 years (62%) than in women older than 50 years (37%).[2]
  - Since the 1960s, incidence rates have decreased in all populations because of Pap smear screening.
- Overall, 5-year relative survival rates are 71%; for localized cervical cancer, they are as high as 92%.[2]

■ Diagnostic Techniques

- Papanicolaou smear
  - The Pap smear was introduced in 1943 to screen for cervical abnormalities.
  - The conventional Pap smear has limitations, including low sensitivity, high false-negative rate, and sampling errors.
- Liquid-based cytology was introduced in the late 1980s.
  - The liquid-based cytology is a more accurate method for detecting cervical abnormalities as compared with the conventional Pap smear.
- Colposcopic exam
  - Colposcopy is used to further evaluate abnormal Pap smears.
  - Colposcopy with guided biopsy detects 69.9% of CIN III lesions.[4]

■ Staging

- Staging of invasive cervical cancer is based on clinical examination and derived from the International Federation of Gynecology and Obstetrics (FIGO) staging system, which was updated in early 2010 (**Table 4.1**).

■ Cervical Intraepithelial Neoplasia (CIN) and HPV

- Approximately 500,000 cases of CIN 2-3 are diagnosed each year in the United States, and about 50–60% are attributable to HPV 16 and HPV 18.[5]
- Low-grade CIN is caused by multiple HPV types.
  - Twenty-five percent is associated with HPV 16 or HPV 18.[6]
  - Five percent is associated with HPV 6 or HPV 11.[7]
- Most low-grade lesions resolve spontaneously with 75% of adults and 90% of adolescents clearing the infections without clinical, surgical, or medical intervention.[8] As a result, the current guidelines do not recommend using HPV testing in the adolescent population.

Table 4.1   International Federation of Gynecology and Obstetrics (FIGO) Staging of Carcinoma of the Cervix Uteri

Stage I   Carcinoma confined to cervix
IA   Invasive carcinoma diagnosed only by microscopy, deepest invasion ≤ 5 mm and largest extension ≥ 7 mm
  IA1   Measured stromal invasion ≤ 3 mm in depth and extension of ≤ 7 mm
  IA2   Measured stromal invasion > 3 mm and ≤ 5 mm with extension of ≤ 7 mm
IB   Visible lesion limited to cervix or preclinical cancer greater than stage IA
  IB1   Visible lesion ≤ 4 cm in greatest dimension
  IB2   Visible lesion > 4 cm in greatest dimension

Stage II   Carcinoma invades beyond uterus, not to pelvic wall or lower third of vagina
IIA   No parametrial invasion
  IIA1   Visible lesion ≤ 4 cm in greatest dimension
  IIA2   Visible lesion > 4 cm in greatest dimension
IIB   Parametrial invasion

Stage III   Tumor extends to pelvic wall and/or involves lower third of vagina and/or causes hydronephrosis or nonfunctioning kidney
IIIA   Tumor involves lower third of vagina, no extension to pelvic wall
IIIB   Extension to pelvic wall and/or hydronephrosis or nonfunctioning kidney

Stage IV   Carcinoma extended beyond true pelvis or involved mucosa bladder or rectum (biopsy proven)
IVA   Spread to adjacent organs
IVB   Spread to distant organs

Source: Adapted from Petru E, Luck H, Stuart G, et al. Gynecologic Cancer Intergroup (GCIG) proposals for changes of the current FIGO staging system. *Eur J Obstet Gynecol Reprod Biol*. 2009;143:69–74.

■ Invasive Cervical Carcinoma and HPV

- The risk of cervical cancer is intimately tied to the type of HPV infection present; nearly all women with cervical cancer have evidence of infection with HPV. There is a more than 400-fold increased risk of cervical cancer if a woman has HPV 16, compared with those not infected with HPV 16.

- Approximately 70% of cervical cancers are caused by HPV types 16 or 18.[9,10]
- HPV 16 accounts for the majority of adenocarcinoma (40%); HPV 18 is found more often in adenocarcinoma (30%) when compared with squamous cell carcinoma.[11]
- Worldwide, HPV 16 can be attributed to 50–60% of squamous cell carcinoma and HPV 18 to 10–15% of squamous cell carcinoma.[12]
- In the United States, screening with the Pap smear led to a decrease in cervical cancer deaths by 74% between 1955 and 1992.[2] The estimated cost of secondary prevention of cervical cancer is $6 billion each year.[13]

■ Screening for Cervical Cancer

- The American Society of Colposcopists and Cytopathologists (ASCCP) released guidance on screening in 2006. These are summarized as follows:[14]
  - For adolescents (age < 20 years)
    - Pap smear screening should begin 3 years after the onset of intercourse or no later than age 21 and annually until age 30.
    - Immunocompromised adolescents should begin screening at initiation of vaginal intercourse.
    - HPV testing is not indicated in adolescents.
    - Pap smear showing atypical squamous cells of unclear significance (ASCUS) or low-grade squamous intraepithelial lesions (L-SIL)
      - Repeat cytology at 12-month intervals for 2 years or if HSIL is found.
      - Colposcopy is indicated if persistence is beyond 2 years or if HSIL is found.
    - Pap smear showing HSIL
      - Colposcopy is indicated.
      - If no CIN 2-3 is found, repeat colposcopy with cytology at 6 month intervals for 2 years.

- If HSIL persists for 2 years without CIN 2-3, diagnostic excisional procedure is indicated.
- If CIN 2-3 is found, manage as per ASCCP guidelines for adolescents.
- Pap smear showing ASCUS
  - Repeat cytology at 6 and 12 months. If high-risk HPV testing was done and is negative, repeat cytology at 12 months. If high-risk HPV testing was positive, colposcopy is indicated.
  - If anything greater than or equal to ASCUS is identified, colposcopy is indicated.
  - If CIN is identified, manage as per ASCCP guidelines.
  - If no CIN is identified, repeat cytology at 12 months or, if high-risk HPV positive, repeat cytology at 6 and 12 months or repeat HPV testing in 12 months.
- Pap smear shows ASCUS, cannot rule out high-grade lesion (also classified as atypical squamous cells–high risk, or ASC-H) or LSIL.
  - Colposcopy is indicated.
  - If CIN 2-3 is not identified, cytology evaluation at 6 and 12 months or HPV testing at 12 months.
  - Routine annual screening after two consecutive normal Pap smears.
  - If any cytologic abnormality greater than or equal to ASC-H is noted or + HPV, colposcopy is again recommended.
- Pap smear shows high-grade squamous intraepithelial lesion (H-SIL)
  - Colposcopy with endocervical sampling is indicated.
  - If no CIN 2-3 is found, colposcopy and cytology at 6-month intervals is recommended for up to 2 years.
  - If HSIL or a high-grade colposcopic lesion persists at any future evaluation, a diagnostic excisional procedure is indicated.
  - If CIN 2-3 is found, manage as per ASCCP guidelines.

- Pap smear shows atypical glandular cells (AGC)
  - Colposcopy with endocervical sampling and high-risk HPV testing is indicated.
  - Endometrial sampling is indicated for anyone over 35 years of age or any woman at risk for endometrial neoplasia regardless of age.
- Findings of cervical intraepithelial neoplasia, grade 1 (CIN 1)[14]
  - Rate of progression to CIN 2 or greater over 2 years is 10% though in the adolescent population it is much lower (3%).
  - Conservative management is recommended with follow-up as per ASCUS/LSIL guidelines.
- CIN 2-3[14]
  - Rate of resolution in adults is 40% and believed to be higher in adolescents.
  - Colposcopy and cytology at 6-month intervals for 2 years or treatment with ablation or excision.
  - If only CIN 2 is noted, observation is preferred.
  - Excisional procedure is recommended if CIN 2-3 persists after 2 years.
- Recently, the American College of Obstetricians and Gynecologists (ACOG) released new screening guidelines based on an evidence-based review. These differ slightly from the 2006 ASCCP guidelines and are summarized as follows:[15]
  - Screening should begin at age 21 years regardless of age onset of intercourse.
  - Cervical cytology screening is recommended every 2 years for women aged 21–29 years.
  - Women older than 30 years with three prior consecutive normal Pap smears may be screened every 3 years.
  - Women who are immunocompromised and have been exposed to diethylstilbestrol (DES) in utero have a higher risk of developing cervical cancer and, hence, may require more frequent screening.
  - Women previously treated for CIN 2-3 or cancer should continue to have annual screenings for 20 years.

- Any attempt at setting an age to discontinue screening must take into account the woman's prior screening history. Typically, the recommended age is 65–70 years.
- Women who have had a total hysterectomy for benign reasons may discontinue Pap smear screening provided there is no history of high-grade CIN.
- Those women with a prior history of CIN 2-3 or an undocumented screening history should continue screening.
- Increasing the interval between Pap smears does not preclude the need for an annual pelvic examination with a gynecologist or primary healthcare professional.

■ Role of HPV Testing

- All of the HPV DNA assays are approved for use with ThinPrep Pap tests.
- HPV testing is used as a triage test in women aged 21 years or older with an ASCUS Pap smear and in postmenopausal women with LSIL Pap smear.
- It may be used as an adjunct to cervical screening in those older than 30 years.
- It should not be used in women younger than 21 years and if positive should not influence management.
- It may be used as a follow-up test after CIN 1 or negative findings on colposcopy in women with prior cytology of ASCUS, ASC-H, LSIL, or AGUS and in follow-up after treatment for CIN 2-3.
- Low-risk women older than 30 years with negative HPV testing and cytology should be rescreened no sooner than 3 years.
- Women who have been vaccinated against HPV 16 or 18 should be screened in the same fashion as those who have not been immunized.
- Hybrid Capture2 HPV DNA Assay detects HPV 16, 18, 31, 33, 35, 39, 45, 51, 52, 56, 58, 59, and 68.
- In March 2009, the U.S. Food and Drug Administration (FDA) approved Cervista HR, which detects those HPV

types identified in the Hybrid Capture 2 as well as HPV 66. Cervista HPV 16/18 detects HPV 16 and 18.

- The FDA-approved indications for Cervista HR are (1) to screen patients with ASCUS cytology to determine the need for colposcopy and (2) to be used with cervical cytology to screen women 30 years or older for high-risk HPV.

- The FDA-approved indications for Cervista HPV 16/18 is for use in women 30 years and older with the Cervista HR test in combination with cytology to detect high-risk HPV types; it may also be used with Cervista HR in patients with ASCUS to detect specific high-risk HPV types. The results of this test are not intended to prevent colposcopy.[16]

- HPV genotyping does not add clinical benefit to the management of women with ASCUS because only approximately 50% of CIN 2+ lesions are associated with HPV 16 or 18.[17]

  - For women 21 years and older with oncogenic HPV-positive ASCUS, the overall 2-year cumulative risk of CIN 2+ was 25%.

  - Stratifying by HPV genotype categories, the cumulative risk of CIN 2+ for women with HPV 16/18–positive ASCUS was approximately 40%, while the risk for women with other oncogenic (non-16/18) HPV-positive ASCUS was approximately 20%.

  - Similar patterns were observed in women aged 21–29 years and women aged 30 years and older.

  - Although HPV genotyping stratified risk to an extent, the risk of CIN 2+ among women with non-16/18 oncogenic HPV-positive ASCUS remained high enough to warrant colposcopy.

  - On the basis of these findings, the 2006 ASCCP guidelines do not recommend the use of HPV genotyping in women with oncogenic HPV-positive ASCUS.

    - Management of women in the general population with ASCUS, who are screened using liquid-based cytology, should have a "reflex" test using a validated assay that detects either 13 or 14 high-risk HPV types.

- If the woman is high-risk HPV DNA positive, she should be referred to colposcopy, even if she tests negative for HPV 16 and HPV 18.[18]

• HPV typing is not recommended for the following:[18]

- Adolescents, defined as women 20 years and younger (regardless of their cytology results)
- Women 21 years and older with ASC-H, LSIL, or HSIL cytology (note: "reflex" HPV testing is acceptable in postmenopausal women with LSIL)
- Routine screening in women before the age of 30 years
- Women considering vaccination against HPV
- Routine sexually transmitted disease screening
- As part of a sexual assault workup
- Women with ASCUS
- As the initial screening test for women 30 years and older

■ Use of HPV genotyping to manage cytology in women older than 30 years[14,19]

• In women older than 30 years with HPV high-risk positive and cytology negative:

- Colposcopy is indicated if HPV 16/18 is positive.
- If HPV 16/18 is negative, repeat both cytology and HPV test at 12 months.
- If both cytology and HPV testing are negative at 12 months, then resume routine screening at 3 years.
- If cytology is negative but HPV is still positive, then colposcopy is indicated.
- If the cytology is abnormal regardless of HPV status, then manage according to ASCCP guidelines.

• In women older than 30 years with negative cytology and HPV negative, perform routine screening in 3 years.

• In women older than 30 years with cytology showing ASCUS or greater, manage as per ASCCP guidelines.

■ Treatment of Cervical Cancer

- Preinvasive disease may be treated with electrocoagulation, cryotherapy, laser ablation, or surgical excision.
  - Cold knife conization removes more cervical tissue than loop excision and better evaluates endocervical extension.
  - Loop excision uses electrocautery, which has caused some concern regarding thermal artifact interfering with pathologic assessment.
  - Cryotherapy is easy to use and inexpensive; however, it does not provide a specimen for pathologic evaluation.
  - Laser ablation is expensive and requires a moderate amount of training.
- Invasive cancer is treated with surgery, radiation, and chemotherapy in selected cases or a combination of these treatment modalities. National Comprehensive Cancer Network (NCCN) 2010 Guidelines are summarized below:[20]
  - Stage IA1 options include
    - Extrafascial hysterectomy
    - Observation if patient desires fertility or if inoperable (only if cone biopsy has negative margins)
    - Modified radical hysterectomy + pelvic lymph node dissection if lymphovascular invasion
  - Stage IA2 options include
    - Radical hysterectomy + pelvic lymph node dissection ± para-aortic lymph node sampling
    - Brachytherapy + pelvic radiation therapy (RT)
    - Radical trachelectomy for fertility preservation + pelvic lymph node dissection ± para-aortic lymph node sampling
  - Stage IB1, IIA (≤ 4 cm) options include
    - Radical hysterectomy + pelvic lymph node dissection + para-aortic lymph node sampling
    - Pelvic RT + brachytherapy
    - Radical trachelectomy for fertility preservation (Stage IB1) + pelvic lymph node dissection ± para-aortic lymph node sampling

- Stage IB2, IIA (> 4 cm) options include
  - Radical hysterectomy + pelvic lymph node dissection + para-aortic lymph node sampling
  - Pelvic RT + concurrent cisplatin-containing chemotherapy + brachytherapy
  - Pelvic RT + concurrent cisplatin-containing chemotherapy + brachytherapy + adjuvant hysterectomy
- Bulky Stage IB2, Stage IIA (> 4 cm), Stages IIB, IIIA, IIIB, IVA
  - Pelvic RT + concurrent cisplatin-containing chemotherapy + brachytherapy

■ References

1. Garcia M, Jemal A, Ward EM, et al. *Global Cancer Facts & Figures 2007*. Atlanta, GA: American Cancer Society; 2007.

2. American Cancer Society. *Cancer Facts & Figures 2009*. Atlanta, GA: American Cancer Society; 2009.

3. Robison K, Dizon DS. *Dx/Rx: Cervical Cancer. Diagnosis and Treatment of Pre-cancerous Lesions (CIN) and Cervical Cancer*. 2nd ed. Sudbury, MA: Jones & Bartlett Learning; 2011:4.

4. Gage JC, Hanson VW, Abbey K, et al. Number of cervical biopsies and sensitivity of colposcopy. *Obstet Gynecol.* 2006;108(2):264–272.

5. Clifford GM, Smith JS, Aguado T, et al. Comparison of HPV type distribution in high-grade cervical lesions and cervical cancer: a meta-analysis. *Br J Cancer.* 2003;89:101–105.

6. The Atypical Squamous Cells of Undetermined Significance/Low-Grade Squamous Intraepithelial Lesions Triage Study (ALTS) Group. Human papillomavirus testing for triage of women with cytologic evidence of low-grade squamous intraepithelial lesions: baseline data from a randomized trial. *J Natl Cancer Inst.* 2000;92:397–402.

7. Herrero R, Castle PE, Schiffman M, et al. Epidemiologic profile of type-specific human papillomavirus infection and cervical neoplasia in Guanacaste, Costa Rica. *J Infect Dis.* 2005;191:1796–1807.

8. Moscicki AB, Shiboski S, Hills NK, et al. Regression of low-grade squamous intraepithelial lesions in young women. *Lancet.* 2004;364:1678–1683.

9. Munoz N, Bosch FX, de Sanjose S, et al. Epidemiologic classification of human papillomavirus types associated with cervical cancer. *N Engl J Med.* 2003;348:518–527.

10. Bosch FX, Manos MM, Munoz N, et al. Prevalence of human papillomavirus in cervical cancer: a worldwide perspective. International Biological Study on Cervical Cancer (IBSCC) Study Group. *J Natl Cancer Inst*. 1995;87:796–802.

11. Castellsagué X, Diaz M, de Sanjose S, et al. Worldwide human papillomavirus etiology of cervical adenocarcinoma and its cofactors: implications for screening and prevention. *J Natl Cancer Inst*. 2006;98:303–315.

12. Clifford GM, Smith JS, Plummer M, et al. Human papillomavirus types in invasive cervical cancer worldwide: a meta-analysis. *Br J Cancer*. 2003;88:63–73.

13. Centers for Disease Control and Prevention. Incidence of Pap test abnormalities within 3 years of a normal Pap test—United States, 1991–1998. *MMWR Morb Mortal Wkly Rep*. 2000;49(44):1001–1003.

14. 2006 consensus guidelines for the management of women with abnormal cervical cancer screening tests. http://www.asccp.org/pdfs/consensus/algorithms_cyto_07.pdf. Accessed October 25, 2009.

15. ACOG practice bulletin: cervical cytology screening. *Obstet Gynecol*. 2009;114:1409–1420.

16. ASCCP HPV clinical update 2009. http://www.asccp.org/pdfs/consensus/clinical_update_20090408.pdf. Accessed October 25, 2009.

17. Smith JS, Lindsay L, Hoots B, et al. Human papillomavirus type distribution in invasive cervical cancer and high-grade cervical lesions: a meta-analysis update. *Int J Cancer*. 2007;121(3):621–632.

18. ASCCP HPV genotyping clinical update 2009. http://www.asccp.org/pdfs/consensus/clinical_update_20090408.pdf. Accessed October 25, 2009.

19. 2009 algorithm: use of HPV genotyping to manage HPV HR * positive/cytology negative women 30 years and older. http://www.asccp.org/pdfs/consensus/hpv_genotyping_20090320.pdf. Accessed October 25, 2009.

20. NCCN clinical practice guidelines in oncology, cervical cancer 2010. http://www.nccn.org/professionals/physician_gls/PDF/cervical.pdf. Accessed May 8, 2010.

CHAPTER 5

HPV and Lower Genital Disease

■ Genital Warts

- An estimated 1 million new cases of genital warts are diagnosed each year.
- Condyloma acuminata are clinically described in 1% of the sexually active population.
  - In women, condyloma are most commonly seen on the vulva, but up to 25% of patients may also have anogenital warts.[1]
  - In men, warts can be located on the urethra, penis, scrotum, and anus.
- Two-thirds of people who have sexual contact with an infected person will develop genital warts.
- The incubation time is approximately 3 months.
- Genital warts are most commonly associated with HPV 6 and 11.
  - Fifty percent of women with genital warts have multiple sites involved.
  - Nielson et al. found that in male external genital samples, the glans/corona, shaft, and scrotum were more likely than anal samples to contain oncogenic HPV (25% vs. 5%). HPV-positive penile shaft and glans/corona samples were also more likely to be infected with multiple HPV types than other sites.[2]
  - Anal intercourse is a risk factor for the development of anogenital warts.
  - Pooling of secretions is thought to be the inciting factor.
- Condyloma, dysplasia, and invasive malignancy can appear similar, making biopsy important in diagnosing genital warts.

- Genital warts may resolve spontaneously, and up to 70% will resolve with treatment. Regardless, they will often recur with or without treatment.
- Condom use may decrease the risk of HPV-associated genital warts. It has been associated with higher rates of regression of cervical dysplasia in women and HPV-associated penile lesions in men.[3]
- There are many treatments options for genital warts (**Table 5.1**).[4,5]
  - Patient-administered therapies include
    - 0.5% Podofilox (Podophyllotoxin, Condylox Watson Pharmaceuticals, Corona, CA)
    - 5% Imiquimod cream (Aldara, Graceway Pharmaceuticals, Bristol, TN)
    - Veregen 15% ointment (Green tea catechins, C.P.M. Contract Pharma GmbH and Co. KG, Feldkirchen-Westerham, Germany)
  - Healthcare professional–administered therapies include
    - 10–25% podophyllin resin
    - 80–90% bichloracetic acid/trichloroacetic acid (BCA/TCA)
    - Cryotherapy
    - Excision
    - Laser vaporization
    - Intralesional interferon
- The goal of treatment is to remove as many visible lesions as noted until the patient's immune system can clear the virus.
- Multiple treatments may be necessary in the immuno-compromised.

■ Vulvar and Vaginal Cancer

- Vulvar and vaginal cancers account for approximately 6% of all gynecologic malignancies.
- 30–35% of vulvar cancers are HPV related.
  - HPV is associated with 70–80% of vulvar dysplasia. HPV 16 is the most common type isolated.

- The precursor lesions to invasive disease is vulvar intraepithelial neoplasia (VIN) and vaginal intraepithelial neoplasia (VAIN). Both are graded I, II, or III on the basis of cellular atypia.
- HPV prevalence is 68% in VIN 1, 85% in VIN 2-3, and 40% in vulvar carcinomas.[6]
- HPV prevalence is 100% for VAIN 1, 90% for VAIN 2-3, and 70% in vaginal carcinomas.[6]
- The annual progression rate of untreated VIN 3 to invasive cancer is at least 10% while CIN 3 progresses at a rate of about 2%. Women with VAIN have a 2% risk of developing invasive cancer.[7,8]

- Unfortunately, there is no routine screening program for these diseases like there is for cervical cancer. Women with visible lesions on the vulvar surface should undergo clinical examination and vulvoscopy if warranted.
- Between 1973 and 2000, the incidence of VIN 3 increased more than 400% in the United States, and the incidence of invasive vulvar cancer increased by 20%.
  - The rate of VIN 3 has also been increasing worldwide and seems to be associated with HPV 16 and HPV 18.[9–12]
- Risk factors for the development of vulvar and vaginal cancer
  - History of vulvar condyloma
  - Tobacco use
  - Immunosuppression
  - History of abnormal Pap smears
  - Increased number of sexual partners
  - Chronic vulvar inflammatory conditions (lichen sclerosis, vulvar dystrophy)
- Vaginal cancer
  - Vaginal cancer is more frequently diagnosed in younger patients, possibly because of HPV.
  - There is a 2.9-fold increase in therapy for genital warts and a 3.8-fold increase in prior abnormal Pap smears in patients with vaginal dysplasia.[13]
    - This is likely due to effects of HPV 16, 18, 31, and 33.[14]

Table 5.1 Topical Treatments for Genital Warts

	Mechanism of Action	Prescribing Instructions	Side Effects	Efficacy
Podofilox 0.5%	Antimitotic agent, destroys warts by stopping cell division at metaphase, inducing tissue local necrosis	Twice daily for 3 consecutive days, with 4 consecutive days of no therapy each week, for a maximum of 4 weeks	Local inflammation, erosions, burning, pain, and itching. Contraindicated for use in the vagina, urethra, perianal area, cervix, and in pregnancy	45–77% clearance 4–38% recurrence
Imiquimod 5%	Immune modifier by inducing cytokines, interferon alpha, tumor necrosis factor, and interleukins	3 times a week, every other day, for up to 16 weeks	Erythema, erosion, itching, skin flaking, and edema. Contraindicated for use on occluded mucus membranes or on the cervix	37–54% clearance 13–19% recurrence
BCA/TCA*	Topical acid	3 times a week for a maximum of 4 weeks.	Ulceration and pain. For use on external skin only. Safe in pregnancy	50–81% response rate High rate of recurrence
Veregen	Sinecatechins reduce expression HPV gene products E6 and E7, which lead to the induction of HPV-induced cell growth and neoplasia. Sinecatechins also may inhibit proinflammatory enzymes and proteases	Up to 250 mg (per application) applied topically, 3 times a day	Erythema, edema, and erosion	50% clearance of wart in 77% patients
10–25% Podophyllin Resin	Antimitotic agent	Apply to external lesions as needed	Nausea, vomiting, fever, confusion, coma, renal failure, ileus, and leukopenia. Contraindicated in pregnancy	20–77% success rate 23–65% recurrence

* Trichloracetic acid

- Vulvar and vaginal dysplasia are diagnosed with biopsy, and treatment is usually local excision. Invasive cancers require more radical surgery and/or chemoradiation.
  - Microinvasive vulvar disease (stromal invasion $\leq$ 1 mm) has minimal risk of lymphatic dissemination and can be treated with wide local excision.
  - Stage I and II vulvar cancers are treated with radical vulvectomy with unilateral or bilateral (if tumor encroaches midline) inguinal lymph node dissection.
  - Stage III and IV vulvar cancers are treated with either radical excision or chemoradiation.
  - Early stage vaginal cancer is treated with either excision or radiation. Advanced vaginal cancer is typically treated with chemoradiation.

Table 5.2   FIGO Staging of Vulvar Cancer

Stage I	Tumor confined to vulva
IA	Lesions $\leq$ 2 cm, stromal invasion $\leq$ 1 mm
IB	Lesions > 2 cm or stromal invasion > 1 mm
Stage II	Any size tumor with extension to adjacent perineal structures (lower third urethra, vagina, anus).
Stage III	Tumor of any size or without extension to adjacent perineal structures with positive inguino-femoral lymph nodes
IIIA	(i) 1 lymph node metastasis ($\geq$ 5 mm) or
	(ii) 1–2 lymph node metastasis(es) (< 5 mm)
IIIB	(i) 2 or more lymph node metastases ($\geq$ 5 mm) or
	(ii) 3 or more lymph node metastases (< 5 mm)
IIIC	Positive nodes with extracapsular spread
Stage IV	Tumor invades other regional (upper 2/3 urethra, upper 2/3 vagina) or distant structures
IVA	(i) Tumor invades upper urethra and/or vaginal mucosa, bladder mucosa, rectal mucosa, or fixed to pelvic bone or
	(ii) Fixed or ulcerated inguino-femoral lymph nodes
IVB	Any distant metastasis, including pelvic lymph nodes

Source: Adapted from Petru E, Luck H, Stuart G, et al. Gynecologic Cancer Intergroup (GCIG) proposals for changes of the current FIGO staging system. *Eur J Obstet Gynecol Reprod Biol*. 2009;143:69–74.

Table 5.3 FIGO Staging of Vaginal Cancer

Stage I	Tumor confined to vaginal mucosa
Stage II	Submucosal infiltration into parametrium, not extending to pelvic wall **IIA** Subvaginal infiltration, not into parametrium **IIB** Parametrial infiltration, not extending to pelvic wall
Stage III	Tumor extending to pelvic wall
Stage IV	
	IVA Tumor invades mucosa of bladder/rectum or extends outside true pelvis **IVB** Distant metastasis

Source: Adapted from Petru E, Luck H, Stuart G, et al. Gynecologic Cancer Intergroup (GCIG) proposals for changes of the current FIGO staging system. *Eur J Obstet Gynecol Reprod Biol*. 2009;143:69–74.

■ Staging of Vulvar and Vaginal Cancer

- Staging of vulvar and vaginal cancers are derived from the International Federation of Gynecology and Obstetrics (FIGO) staging system, which was updated in early 2010 (**Table 5.2** and **Table 5.3**).

■ References

1. Handley JM, Maw RD, Lawther H, et al. Human papillomavirus DNA detection in primary anogenital warts and cervical low-grade intraepithelial neoplasias in adults by in situ hybridization. *Sex Transm Dis*. 1992;19:225–229.
2. Nielson CM, Flores R, Harris RB, et al. Human papillomavirus prevalence and type distribution in male anogenital sites and semen. *Cancer Epidemiol Biomarkers Prev*. 2007; 16:1107–1114.
3. Holmes KK, Levine R, Weaver M. Effectiveness of condom in preventing sexually transmitted infections. *Bull World Health Organ*. 2004;84:454–461.
4. Monk BJ, Tewari KS. The spectrum and clinical sequelae of human papillomavirus infection. *Gynecol Oncol*. 2007; 107(suppl):S6–S13.

5. Mayeaux E, Dunton C. Modern management of external genital warts. *J Low Genit Tract Dis.* 2008;12(3):185–192.

6. De Vuyst H, Clifford GM, Nascimento MC, et al. Prevalence and type distribution of human papillomavirus in carcinoma and intraepithelial neoplasia of the vulva, vagina and anus: a meta-analysis. *Int J Cancer.* 2009;124(7):1626–1636.

7. Jones RW. Vulvar intraepithelial neoplasia: current perspectives. *Eur J Gynaecol Oncol.* 2001;22:393–402.

8. Dodge JA, Eltabbakh GH, Mount SL, et al. Clinical features and risk of recurrence among patients with vaginal intraepithelial neoplasia. *Gynecol Oncol.* 2001;83:363–369.

9. Judson PL, Habermann EB, Baxter NN, et al. Trends in the incidence of invasive and in situ vulvar carcinoma. *Obstet Gynecol.* 2006;107:1018–1022.

10. Joura EA, Losch A, Haider-Angeler MG, et al. Trends in vulvar neoplasia. Increasing incidence of vulvar intraepithelial neoplasia and squamous cell carcinoma of the vulva in young women. *J Reprod Med.* 2000;45:613–615.

11. Jones RW, Baranyai J, Stables S. Trends in squamous cell carcinoma of the vulva: the influence of vulvar intraepithelial neoplasia. *Obstet Gynecol.* 1997;90:448–452.

12. Hillemanns P, Wang X. Integration of HPV-16 and HPV-18 DNA in vulvar intraepithelial neoplasia. *Gynecol Oncol.* 2006;100:276–282.

13. Brinton LA, Nasca PC, Mallin K, et al. Case-control study of *in situ* and invasive carcinoma of the vagina. *Gynecol Oncol.* 1990;38:49–54.

14. Reeves WC, Brinton LA, Garcia M, et al. Human papillomavirus infection and cervical cancer in Latin America. *N Engl J Med.* 1989;320:1437–1441.

CHAPTER 6

HPV and Head and Neck Cancer

- Oropharyngeal carcinomas comprise tumors that arise from the lip, oral cavity, oropharynx, hypopharynx, nasopharynx, glottic and supraglottic larynx, sinuses, and salivary glands.
  - HPV infection is specifically tied to an increased risk of tumors arising in the oropharynx and specifically arising in the palatine and lingual tonsils.
- In the United States in 2009, there were 35,720 new cases of oropharyngeal cancers in both sexes and 7,600 estimated deaths.[1]
- Although tobacco and alcohol have typically been identified as risk factors, HPV is now recognized as another major source of risk. In fact, 24% of oropharynx cancer cases are HPV related in both sexes.
  - HPV 16 and 18 are the causative types of 89–95% of oropharynx and mouth cancers.
- The epithelia of the tonsil and tongue base are characterized by cryptic invaginations that expose basal epithelial cells, which HPV preferentially infects. This unique structural aspect might predispose oropharyngeal tissue to infection, leading to the higher rates of HPV disease here as compared with the oral cavity, which is covered by thicker stratified squamous mucosa.[2]
- Method of transmission
  - In a study of patients with head and neck squamous cancer, those with no oral sexual partners had no increased risk of having HPV in their tumor compared with a twofold risk in those with one to five lifetime oral sex partners and a fivefold risk for those with more than six lifetime oral sexual partners.[3]
- HPV appears to be a prognostic factor for oropharyngeal cancer (**Table 6.1**). In a prospective cohort of 96 Stage

Table 6.1 Differences Between HPV-Negative and -Positive Oropharyngeal Carcinoma

	HPV Negative	HPV Positive
Molecular Factors	p53 mutational loss common	p53 wild-type present
	Rb upregulated	Rb downregulated
	p16 underexpression	p16 overexpression
	D cyclin overexpression	D cyclin underexpressed
	No HPV DNA/RNA	HPV DNA (type 16 in > 85% of cases)
		HPV E6 and E7 RNA
Epidemiological Factors	Heavy smoking	Never smoked
	Heavy alcohol	Mild/moderate alcohol
	Low marijuana exposure	High marijuana exposure
	Poor dentition	Intact dentition
	Low oral sex exposure	High oral sex exposure
	Older age (> 50 years)	Younger age (< 45 years)
	Lower socioeconomic status	Higher socioeconomic status
	Decreasing incidence	Increasing incidence
Clinical Factors	All head and neck sites	Predominantly oropharynx (tonsil and tongue base)
	Worse survival	Better survival
	Radiation response unpredictable	More radiosensitive

Source: Adapted from Gillespie MB, Rubinchik S, Hoel B, et al. Human papillomavirus and oropharyngeal cancer: what you need to know in 2009. *Curr Treat Options Oncol.* September 19, 2009.

III and Stage IV oropharyngeal and laryngeal cancer patients treated with combination chemotherapy and radiation, patients with tumors positive for HPV DNA had improved 2-year overall survival (95% vs. 62%) compared with HPV-negative patients.[4]

- HPV positivity may lower the risk of overall mortality by 28% and disease recurrence by 49%.[2]

■ Early diagnosis of oral mucosal lesions has recently been advocated as a method to improve cancer detection and treatment for oropharyngeal cancers.

- The utilization of an oral chemolumenoscopy system, coupled with TBlue Oral Marking System (Vizilite, Zila Pharmaceuticals), has been reported in a multicenter trial to be effective in identifying possible abnormal mucosal lesions, which then can be stained and mapped on a mouth diagram.

- Detailed oral screening and referral for further evaluation, including possible biopsies, may also be advocated.

- Screening may be considered in high-risk populations for those who may be at increased risk for oral abnormalities.

■ Staging is critical at presentation and is the most important predictor of survival.

- The American Joint Committee on Cancer (AJCC) Staging System is used for staging oropharyngeal carcinoma (**Table 6.2**).

■ Treatment very much depends on stage of disease.

- Surgical therapy remains the principle modality of treatment of oropharyngeal cancers.

- Radiation or chemoradiation can be used for locally advanced (Stage III) disease following surgery.

  ■ RTOG 73-03 was a trial evaluating the optimal sequence of radiation and surgery.[5] In this trial, radiation was given either preoperatively or postoperatively in patients with operable but advanced disease. Of 277 evaluable patients, significantly better local control was achieved, though no effect in overall survival was seen.

Table 6.2 **American Joint Commission on Cancer (AJCC) Staging System for Oropharyngeal Cancers**

Stage	T	N	M
0	Tis	0	0
1	1	0	0
II	2	0	0
III	3	0	0
	1–3	1	0
IVA	4a	0–1	0
	1–3	2	0
	4a	2	0
IVB	4b	Any	0
	Any	3	0
IVC	Any	Any	1

Tumor	Tx	Tumor cannot be assessed.
	T0	No evidence of primary tumor.
	T1	Tumor 2 cm or less
	T2	Tumor > 2 but < 4 cm
	T3	Tumor > 4 cm or extends to lingual surface of epiglottis
	T4a	Invasion to the larynx, tongue, medial pterygoid, hard palate or mandible
	T4b	Invasion of lateral pterygoid muscle, pterygoid plates, lateral nasopharynx, skull base, or encasement of the carotid artery.
Nodes	Nx	Nodes cannot be assessed.
	N0	No regional node metastases.
	N1	Metastases in a single ipsilateral node, 3 cm or less in greatest dimension
	N2	Metastases in single ipsilateral node, > 3 cm but < 6 cm; or in multiple ipsilateral nodes, none > 6 cm; or in bilateral or contralateral nodes, none > 6 cm.
	N3	Metastases in a lymph node > 6 cm in greatest dimension.
Metastasis	M0	No distant metastases
	M1	Distant metastases present

Source: Adapted from *AJCC Cancer Staging Manual*. 7th ed. New York, NY: Springer New York Inc; 2010.

■ References

1. American Cancer Society. *Cancer Facts & Figures 2009.* Atlanta, GA: American Cancer Society; 2009.

2. Gillespie MB, Rubinchik S, Hoel B, et al. Human papillomavirus and oropharyngeal cancer: what you need to know in 2009. *Curr Treat Options Oncol.* September 19, 2009.

3. Gillison ML, D'Souza G, Westra W, et al. Distinct risk factor profiles for human papillomavirus type 16-positive and human papillomavirus type 16-negative head and neck cancers. *J Natl Cancer Inst.* 2008;100:407–420.

4. Fakhry C, Westra W, Li S, et al. Improved survival of patients with human papillomavirus-positive head and neck squamous cell carcinoma in a prospective clinical trial. *J Natl Cancer Inst.* 2008;100:261–269.

5. Tupchong L, Scott CB, Blitzer PH, et al. Randomized study of preoperative versus postoperative radiation therapy in advanced head and neck carcinoma: long term follow-up of RTOG study 73-03. *Int J Radiat Oncol Biol Phys.* 1991;20:21–8.

HPV and Anal Cancer

- Squamous cell cancer of the anus accounts for only 1.5% of all gastrointestinal cancers in the United States.[1]
- In 2009, there were an estimated 5290 new cases and 710 deaths from anorectal cancer in the United States.[2]
- Eighty percent of anal cancers are HPV related in both sexes.
  - Ninety-two percent of anal cancers are HPV 16/18 related.
  - Ninety percent of anogenital warts in the United States are caused by HPV 6 and 11.[3]
  - HPV (most commonly 6 and 11) is found in approximately 90% of anal dysplasia and anal carcinoma in situ.[4] AIN is often found incidentally at time of hemorrhoidectomy or excision of perianal warts.
- Risk factors are multifactorial.[5]
  - History of persistent high-risk genotype HPV infection
  - Infection with multiple HPV genotypes
  - Cervical dysplasia or cancer
    - Women with cervical HPV infection have been shown to have greater than a threefold increased risk of concurrent anal infection.[6]
  - HIV seropositivity
  - Low CD4 count
  - Cigarette smoking
  - Anoreceptive intercourse
  - Immunosuppression following solid organ transplant
  - Condom use
    - Studies have shown any condom use is associated with anal HPV acquisition, while use more than 50% of the time is associated with a protective effect.[7]

Table 7.1   AJCC Staging for Anal Cancer

Primary Tumor (T)	
TX	Primary tumor cannot be assessed
T0	No evidence of primary tumor
Tis	Carcinoma in situ (Bowen's disease, high-grade squamous intraepithelial lesion (HSIL), anal intraepithelial neoplasia II-III (AIN II-III))
T1	Tumor $\leq$ 2 cm in greatest dimension
T2	Tumor > 2 cm but not > 5 cm in greatest dimension
T3	Tumor > 5 cm in greatest dimension
T4	Tumor of any size invades adjacent organ(s) (vagina, urethra, bladder)
Regional Lymph Nodes (N)	
NX	Regional lymph nodes cannot be assessed
N0	No regional lymph node metastasis
N1	Metastasis in perirectal lymph node(s)
N2	Metastasis in unilateral internal iliac and/or inguinal lymph node(s)
N3	Metastasis in perirectal and inguinal lymph nodes and/or bilateral internal iliac and/or inguinal lymph nodes
Distant Metastasis (M)	
M0	No distant metastasis
M1	Distant metastasis

Source: Adapted from *AJCC Cancer Staging Manual*. 7th ed. New York, NY: Springer New York Inc; 2010.

- The association between condom use and anal HPV acquisition may be because of using the same condom for vaginal intercourse followed by anal intercourse.
- There is no recommended protocol to screen for anal dysplasia, and the value of anal cytology remains controversial, hence further study is warranted.
  - There is a reported sensitivity of 83% and a specificity of 38% for AIN, which is comparable with that reported for cervical cytology.[8]
- Staging for anal cancer is described in **Table 7.1**.
- Depending on extent of disease, treatment can encompass a combination of concurrent chemotherapy and radiation and/or surgery.

■ References

1. Monk B, Tewari K. The spectrum and clinical sequelae of human papillomavirus infection. *Gynecol Oncol.* 2007;107(suppl):S6–S13.

2. American Cancer Society. *Cancer Facts & Figures 2009.* Atlanta, GA: American Cancer Society; 2009.

3. Greer CE, Wheeler CM, Ladner MB, et al. Human papillomavirus (HPV) type distribution and serological response to HPV type 6 virus-like particles in patients with genital warts. *J Clin Microbiol.* 1995;33:2058–2063.

4. De Vuyst H, Clifford GM, Nascimento MC, et al. Prevalence and type distribution of human papillomavirus in carcinoma and intraepithelial neoplasia of the vulva, vagina and anus: a meta-analysis. *Int J Cancer.* 2009;124(7):1626–1636.

5. Uronis HE, Bendell JC. Anal cancer: an overview. *Oncologist.* 2007;12:524–534.

6. Hernandez BY, McDuffie K, Zhu X, et al. Anal human papillomavirus infection in women and its relationship with cervical infection. *Cancer Epidemiol Biomarkers Prev.* 2005;14:2550–2556.

7. Nielson C, Harris R, Dunne E, et al. Risk factors for anogenital human papillomavirus infection in men. *J Infect Dis.* 2007;196:1137–1145.

8. Fox PA, Seet JE, Stebbing J, et al. The value of anal cytology and human papillomavirus typing in the detection of anal intraepithelial neoplasia: a review of cases from an anoscopy clinic. *Sex Transm Infect.* 2005;81:142–146.

CHAPTER 8

HPV and Penile Cancer

- In 2009, there were an estimated 1290 new cases and 300 deaths from penile cancer.[1]
- Risk factors for penile cancer include HPV 16/18 infection, chronic irritation, socioeconomic factors, phimosis, and smoking.[2]
  - Epidemiologic evidence suggests that childhood circumcision may reduce the risk.
  - In one study, no differences in the acquisition of HPV infection was noted in a cohort of 357 men followed for more than a year.[3] However, the duration of infection was significantly longer in uncircumcised men, suggesting that circumcision may protect men by speeding up resolution of infection.
- Nodal metastases are common, but distant metastases rarely occurs.[4]
- Sixty-three percent of penile cancers are HPV 16/18 related but subtypes 6, 11, 16, and 31 have also been commonly seen.[5,6] Global HPV prevalence in one study was estimated at 47%. Relative contribution for the subtypes was HPV 16 (60.23%), HPV 18 (13.35%), HPV 6/11 (8.13%), HPV 31 (1.16%), HPV 45 (1.16%), HPV 33 (0.97%), HPV 52 (0.58%), and other types (2.47%).[7]
- There is a clear peak in penile HPV prevalence in men younger than 30 years, followed by a steep decrease in the 30s, but then it increases steadily until age 60 years. This increasing prevalence of penile HPV could explain why women at an older age are still exposed to HPV.[8]
- Penile cancer staging is shown in **Table 8.1**.
- Treatment is typically conservative for early stage disease (laser, cryotherapy, topical agents, local excision) and

Table 8.1   Staging for Penile Cancer

	Primary Tumor/Nodal and Distant Metastasis
Tx	Primary tumor cannot be assessed
T0	No evidence of primary tumor
Tis	Carcinoma in situ
Ta	Noninvasive verrucous carcinoma (broad pushing penetration/invasion allowed)
T1a	Tumor invades subepithelial connective tissue without lymphovascular invasion (LVI) and is not poorly differentiated
T1b	Tumor invades subepithelial connective tissue with LVI or is poorly differentiated
T2	Tumor invades corpus spongiosum or cavernosum
T3	Tumor invades urethra
T4	Tumor invades other adjacent structures
Nx	Regional nodes cannot be assessed
N0	No palpable or visibly enlarged inguinal nodes
N1	Palpable mobile unilateral inguinal node
N2	Palpable mobile multiple or bilateral inguinal nodes
N3	Palpable fixed inguinal nodal mass or pelvic lymphadenopathy unilateral or bilateral
M0	No distant metastasis
M1	Distant metastasis

Source: Adapted from: *AJCC Cancer Staging Manual.* 7th ed. New York, NY: Springer New York Inc; 2010.

more radical for advanced disease (partial/complete amputation, chemotherapy, radiation therapy) and includes evaluation of inguinal lymph nodes.

- Surgical therapy can consist of organ-sparing surgery to total penectomy, depending on involvement.

- Bhagat et al. looked at factors that may predict inguinal node involvement from penile cancer by evaluating 106 patients seen at their program in India.[9] They found that high tumor grade ($p = 0.004$), lymphovascular space invasion ($p = 0.01$), and palpable inguinal adenopathy ($p = 0.05$) predicted nodal involvement.

- For patients with squamous cell carcinoma confined to the gland, postoperative brachytherapy was shown to be a highly effective conservation treatment.[10] In one trial, 144 patients were treated, in whom fewer than 20% had undergone inguinal node dissection. Long-term cancer-specific survival was 92%, and the diameter of the primary tumor was found to increase significantly the risk of tumor recurrence. Following brachytherapy, however, the rate of painful ulceration or stenosis was 26% and 29%, respectively.

- Close surveillance is recommended for three groups of patients:[11]
  - Men treated with phallus-sparing surgery (e.g., laser ablation, topical treatment, or primary radiation)
  - Those with clinically negative nodes and managed with primary excision but without lymphadenectomy, whose pathology returns with high-risk tumors (pT2-3, grade 3, presence of lymphovascular involvement)
  - Those with nodal metastases after primary lymphadenectomy.

- Chemotherapy has a limited role in treating recurrent, advanced, or metastatic disease and is not curative.[12]
  - One potential modality with promise is the intraarterial delivery of chemotherapy (IAC). Chen et al. reported the experience of five patients treated with IAC in Japan.[13] Five patients received a drug

combination of methotrexate, mitomycin C, bleomycin, cisplatin, and etoposide, with all reported to have responded (1 complete, 4 partial). Three of the four partial responders underwent partial penectomy, suggesting downstaging of tumor is possible. The long-term results of IAC have yet to be delineated.

■ References

1. Jemal A., Siegel R, Ward E, et al. Cancer statistics, 2009. *CA Cancer J Clin*. 2009;59:225–249.

2. Watson RA. Human papillomavirus: confronting the epidemic—a urologist's perspective. *Rev Urol*. 2005;7:135–144.

3. Hernandez BY, Shvetsov YB, Goodman MT, et al. Reduced clearance of penile human papillomavirus infection in uncircumcised men. *J Infect Dis*. 2010;201:1340–1343.

4. Pizzocaro G, Piva L, Bandieramonte G, Tana, S. Up-to-date management of carcinoma of the penis. *Eur Urol*. 1997;32:5–15.

5. O'Brien WM, Jenson AB, Lancaster WD, Maxted WC. Human papillomavirus typing of penile condyloma. *J Urol*. 1989;141:863–865.

6. Nielson CM, Flores R, Harris RB, et al. Human papillomavirus prevalence and type distribution in male anogenital sites and semen. *Cancer Epidemiol Biomarkers Prev*. 2007;16:1107–1114.

7. Miralles-Guri C, Bruni L, Cubilla AL, et al. Human papillomavirus prevalence and type distribution in penile carcinoma. *J Clin Pathol*. 2009;62:870–878.

8. Castellsagué X, Schneider A, Kaufmann AM, Bosch FX. HPV vaccination against cervical cancer in women above 25 years of age: key considerations and current perspectives. *Gynecol Oncol*. 2009;115(suppl):S15–S23.

9. Bhagat SK, Gopalakrishnan G, Kekre NS, et al. Factors predicting inguinal node metastasis in squamous cell cancer of penis. *World J Urol*. 2010;28:93–98.

10. de Crevoisier R, Slimane K, Sanfilippo N, et al. Long-term results of brachytherapy for carcinoma of the penis confined to the glans (N- or NX). *Int J Radiat Oncol Biol*. 2009;74:1150–1156.

11. Sánchez-Ortiz RF, Pettaway CA. Natural history, management, and surveillance of recurrent squamous cell penile carcinoma: a risk-based approach. *Urol Clin North Am*. 2003;30:853–867.

12. Protzel C, Ruppin S, Milerski S, Klebingat K, Hakenberg OW. [The current state of the art of chemotherapy of penile cancer: results of a nationwide survey of German clinics]. *Urologe A.* 2009;48:1495–1498.

13. Chen C, Kang C, Chiang P. Intra-arterial infusion of chemotherapy in the treatment of penile cancer. *Jpn J Clin Oncol.* 2009;39:825–828.

CHAPTER 9

Preventing Infection: The HPV Vaccine

■ Background[1]

- It is estimated that the vaccine will prevent 50% of high-grade precancerous lesions and 66% of invasive cancers.[2]
- Gardasil, a quadrivalent vaccine manufactured by Merck, contains antigens for HPV types 6, 11, 16, and 18. Cervarix, a bivalent vaccine manufactured by GlaxoSmithKline, contains antigens for HPV 16 and HPV 18. Neither vaccine contains thimerosal or antibiotics.
- The HPV L1 protein, the antigen in both vaccines, is produced using recombinant techniques. These virus-like particles are identical to HPV virions morphologically but lack the viral DNA core.
- The vaccines induce a virus-neutralizing antibody response against L1 and L2 without posing an infectious or oncogenic risk. In contrast to natural infection, vaccination is highly immunogenic, activating both humoral and cellular immune responses. Immune responses after natural infection are not always protective against reinfection, and the duration of natural immunity is unknown.[3]

■ Vaccine Administration (Table 9.1)

- In the United States, only females are vaccinated; however, in Australia and in Europe, males are also vaccinated.
- Ideally, the vaccine should be administered before the first episode of sexual intercourse as most HPV infections are acquired within the first few months after sexual debut.

Table 9.1   Summary of American Cancer Society (ACS) Recommendations for Human Papilloma Virus (HPV) Vaccine Use to Prevent Cervical Cancer and Its Precursors

- Routine HPV vaccination is recommended for females aged 11–12 years.

- Females as young as age 9 years may receive HPV vaccination.

- HPV vaccination is also recommended for females aged 13–18 years to catch up missed vaccine or to complete the vaccination series.

- There are currently insufficient data to recommend for or against universal vaccination of females aged 19–26 years in the general population. A decision about whether a woman aged 19–26 years should receive the vaccine should be based on an informed discussion between the woman and her healthcare provider regarding her risk of previous HPV exposure and potential benefit from vaccination. Ideally the vaccine should be administered before potential exposure to genital HPV through sexual intercourse because the potential benefit is likely to diminish with increasing number of lifetime sexual partners.

- HPV vaccination is not currently recommended for women older than age 26 years or for males.

- Screening for cervical intraepithelial neoplasia and cancer should continue in both vaccinated and unvaccinated women according to current ACS early detection guidelines.

Source: Adapted from the ACS, *CA Cancer J Clin. 2007;57:7–28.*

- In the United States, 6.2% of adolescents have sexual intercourse before 13 years of age, and the median age at first intercourse is 16 to 17 years.[4]
- The Advisory Committee on Immunization Practices recommends routine vaccination of girls 11 to 12 years of age and "catch-up" vaccination of girls and young women 13 to 26 years of age.[5]

- The vaccine may be administered to immunocompromised individuals especially because they are at higher risk of developing sequelae from HPV infection.

- The vaccine should not be administered to acutely ill females, to women with hypersensitivity reactions to yeast, or to pregnant females.

- It is not necessary to test females for HPV 16 or 18 before vaccination as most women will not be infected with both types at the same time. Similarly, vaccination is acceptable in women with abnormal Pap smears or genital warts as it is unlikely that a female will be infected with all vaccine-targeted HPV types.

- The quadrivalent vaccine is given at 0, 2, and 6 months while the bivalent vaccine is administered at 0, 1, and 6 months.

- It is unknown whether the vaccines will confer lifelong immunity or whether booster vaccines will be necessary.

Mechanism of Action

- The antigens in the both bivalent and quadrivalent HPV vaccines are naked icosohedral virus-like particles (VLPs) composed of the major HPV virion protein L1.

- Vaccine protection is largely due to production of antibodies. Antibodies work by preventing binding of virus to the cell surface/basement membrane and by preventing virus conformational changes needed for entry into the cell.

- Vaccination generates high concentrations of neutralizing antibodies to L1, and vaccination may provide protection against HPV infection through neutralization of virus by serum IgG.

- Antibodies function in two ways to protect against HPV infection. First, serum antibodies are transudated into genital tract mucus. Second, HPV infection requires trauma that exposes the epithelial basement membrane to the virus resulting in direct exudation of systemic antibodies at the site of virus infection.[6,7]

- Vaccination is better than natural immunity.
  - All females seroconverted in vaccine trials as compared with 54–69% by natural immunity.
  - With natural immunity, there is no viremia, resulting in poor access of the virus to lymph nodes.
  - The vaccine is delivered rapidly in virus-like particles to blood and lymph nodes leading to a T-helper cell and B-cell response.

■ Clinical Activity

- Both vaccines have shown 90% efficacy in preventing CIN 2, CIN 3, and adenocarcinoma in situ caused by HPV 16 or HPV 18 among women not infected with those HPV types.[8–15]

- In a cohort representing the general population (women with a possible prior exposure to HPV), at 35 months efficacy for the quadrivalent vaccine against CIN 2-3 was 30–33% regardless of the HPV type identified in the lesion. Vaccine efficacy against CIN 2 or greater associated with only HPV 16 or 18 was 93%.[16]
  - In HPV-naïve women, vaccine efficacy was 70% for CIN 2 and 87% for CIN 3 regardless of the HPV type identified in the lesion.
  - Although vaccine protection is most important for HPV 16 and 18 in terms of cancer prevention, efficacy against CIN 2 or greater for 12 nonvaccine oncogenic types is 54%. Most commonly protected against was HPV 31 (closely related to HPV 16) and HPV 45 (closely related to HPV 18). Cross-protection was also noted for HPV 33.

- In the bivalent vaccine, preventive efficacy against HPV 16 or HPV 18 was 94.4% at 42 months.[15]

- Seroconversion rates were 97.5% or greater in multiple studies of both the bivalent and quadrivalent vaccine.[8–11]

- There was a strong amnestic response to antigen challenge 5 years after vaccination with the quadrivalent vaccine consistent with long-lasting protection.[17]

- The vaccine does not protect women already infected with HPV 16 or 18 at the time of vaccination.[9,12]

- The HPV vaccine protection extends beyond cervical cancer. The quadrivalent vaccine is 97–100% effective in preventing VIN 2-3 or VAIN 2-3 caused by HPV 16 or 18 in HPV 16/18–naïve women. It is 71% effective in the prevention of VIN/VAIN 2-3 in a population of women with prevaccine HPV.[13]

- A decrease in the number of colposcopies and cervical excisional procedures has been seen after vaccination, which could impact rates of preterm birth and other adverse pregnancy outcomes.

■ Quadrivalent Vaccine (Table 9.2)

- Gardasil (Merck) is an L1-based vaccine.

- The quadrivalent vaccine costs approximately $375 for the entire series and is covered by some health insurers.[18]

- The quadrivalent HPV vaccine was approved in June 2006 by the U.S. Food and Drug Administration (FDA), and the indication for its use was expanded in September 2008. The vaccine is indicated for women between 9 and 26 years of age for preventing
  - Cervical, vulvar, and vaginal cancer caused by HPV 16 or HPV 18.
  - Genital warts caused by HPV 6 or HPV 11.
  - Lesions caused by HPV types 6, 11, 16, or 18 (CIN 1, CIN 2, and CIN 3; cervical adenocarcinoma in situ; and vulvar or vaginal intraepithelial neoplasia grades 2 and 3).[19]

- The vaccine efficacy against VIN 2-3 and VAIN 2-3 was 100% in the according-to-protocol group and 71% in the modified-intention-to-treat group.[13]

Table 9.2 Comparison of Cervarix and Gardasil

	Cervarix	Gardasil
HPV Types	16, 18	16, 18, 6, 11
Production System	Insect cells infected with recombinant baculovirus	Yeast
Adjuvant	ASO4 (aluminium salt + MPL (3-O-desacyl-4'-monophosphoryl lipid A))	Alum
Diseases Protected Against	Anogenital cancers, including cervical, vulvar, vaginal, and anal cancers and their associated precursor lesions (and a subset of head and neck cancers)	Anogenital cancers, including cervical, vulvar, vaginal, and anal cancers and their associated precursor lesions (and a subset of head and neck cancers), genital warts, and laryngeal papillomas
Length of Protection	5.5 years	At least 5 years
Dose	0.5 mL dose containing 20 μg HPV 16 L1 and 20 μg HPV 18 L1	0.5 mL dose containing 20 μg HPV 6 L1, 40 μg HPV 11 L1, 40 μg HPV 16 L1 and 20 μg HPV18 L1
Recommended Administration	Three intramuscular injections at 0, 1, and 6 months	Three intramuscular injections at 0, 2, and 6 months
Recommended Age Group for Vaccination	10–25 years	9–26 years
Cost ($US)	$100/dose	$120/dose

Source: Adapted from Monie A, Hung CF, Roden R, Wu TC. Cervarix: a vaccine for the prevention of HPV 16, 18-associated cervical cancer. Biologics. 2008;2(1):97–105.

- Vaccine efficacy is not affected by current or past exposure to one of the vaccine HPV types. In a combined analysis of FUTURE I and II, women with evidence of current or past infection with one or more of the vaccine types still demonstrated 100% efficacy in the prevention of CIN 2-3 or AIS associated with vaccine types to which the vaccinee had no prior evidence of exposure.[20]
- Gardisil is approved for boys aged 9–15 years in the European Union.

■ Bivalent Vaccine

- Cervarix (GlaxoSmithKline) has been approved in Europe and Australia and was approved on October 16, 2009, by the FDA for use in the United States.
- Cervarix is a L1 vaccine that targets HPV 16 and 18.
- The expected cost is $100 per dose.
- The recommended age of vaccination is 10–25 years of age.
- The vaccine has shown an efficacy of 90% against CIN 2 or greater in lesions containing HPV 16 and 18.[10]
- In one study, mean titers of serum-neutralizing antibodies were 2.3–4.8-fold higher for HPV 16 and 6.8–9.1 times higher for HPV 18 after vaccination with Cervarix as compared with Gardasil. Anti–HPV 16 and 18 antibodies were also higher in cervicovaginal secretions in the Cervarix cohort. The clinical significance of this is unknown.[21]
- Cross-protection with HPV 31 and 45 has been demonstrated, which results in protection against 80% of cervical cancers. The duration of cross-protection may be less than that for HPV 16 and 18.[15]
- The vaccine has been shown to be effective over a 5-year period.[15]
- In a Phase III trial, higher antibody levels were noted in preteens/adolescents as compared with women aged 15–25 years.[22] Similarly, Gardasil has been shown to induce higher antibody responses in the 10- to 15-year-old age group as compared with the 16- to 23-year-olds.[8] For an optimal effect, it is best to vaccinate adolescents at an age before sexual debut.

■ Women Older Than Age 25 Years

- The vaccine is safe in all age groups.
- Although the risk of acquiring a new HPV infection peaks during the third decade, sexually active women of all ages continue to be at risk.
  - In the United States, HPV prevalence is more than 15% in the 26 years and older age group and more than 10% in the 30 years and older age group.[23]
  - In a retrospective study in Nottingham, women aged 21, 31, 41, and 51 years had comparable 3-year acquisition rates of HPV 16 and 18 (3.7–3% for HPV 16 and 5.3–3.8% for HPV 18).[24]
- Studies have indicated persistent HPV infection increases with age. In a population-based cohort study in Costa Rica over a median interval of 5 years, the trend was stronger for persistence of HPV 16: 15% for women < 25 years, 25% for women aged 25–34 years; 27% for women aged 35–44 years; 42% for women aged 45–64 years; and 70% for women ≥ 65 years.[25] This persistence puts older women at continued risk for developing cervical cancer.
- Immunogenicity data for the bivalent vaccine shows that women up to age 55 years develop strong HPV 16 and 18 antibody responses. Titers in the 46- to 55-year-old age group are eightfold higher than those associated with natural immunity in the 15- to 25-year-old age group.[26]
- The quadrivalent vaccine has also been evaluated in an older cohort of women aged 24–45 years. It is efficacious, but less so than that seen in women younger than 26 years, possibly because of the increased incidence of HPV in the younger population.[27]
  - In the HPV-naïve cohort, the quadrivalent vaccine was 90.5% efficacious against HPV 6, 11, 16, and 18 and 83% efficacious against HPV 16 and 18 only.
  - When women with a history of HPV are included, the efficacy was 31% for HPV 6, 11, 16, and 18 as compared with 21.6% for HPV 16 and 18.

■ Safety/Adverse Events

■ Pain, erythema, swelling at the injection site, headache, fatigue, and myalgia are reported side effects of the quadrivalent vaccine. Rates of serious adverse events were not higher among recipients of vaccine as compared with placebo for either vaccine.[10,12,28]

■ Two-and-a-half years later, 772 reports (6.2% of all reports) described serious adverse effects following immunization. The reporting rates per 100,000 quadrivalent HPV doses distributed were 8.2 for syncope; 7.5 for local site reactions; 6.8 for dizziness; 5.0 for nausea; 4.1 for headache; 3.1 for hypersensitivity reactions; 2.6 for urticaria; 0.2 for venous thromboembolic events, autoimmune disorders, and Guillain-Barré syndrome; 0.1 for anaphylaxis and death; 0.04 for transverse myelitis and pancreatitis; and 0.009 for motor neuron disease.[29]

■ There are no controlled trials in pregnant women, and HPV vaccination is not recommended in this population of women.

■ The efficacy of the vaccine in men has been investigated.
  • The immunologic response to the quadrivalent vaccine in boys is equivalent to that in girls. Preliminary data suggest that the quadrivalent vaccine is effective in preventing HPV infection and HPV-related anogenital disease among uninfected young men.[8,11,30,31]
  • Giuliano and Palefsky presented updated results of a randomized clinical trial of the quadrivalent vaccine in young men.[32] The trial consisted of 3463 heterosexual men (HM) aged 16 to 23 years and 602 men who had sex with men (MSM) aged 16 to 26 years. Criteria for entry included having no prior evidence of genital warts or lesions, fewer than five lifetime sexual partners, and HIV negativity. With 24 months of follow-up, the HM cohort showed that vaccine efficacy against HPV-related genital lesions was 98% (for HPV 6/16), 97% (for HPV 18), and 99% (for HPV 11); vaccination was associated with an 86% reduction in persistent HPV infection; and it was 100% effective

against the development of penile intraepithelial neoplasia. In the MSM cohort, the efficacy of vaccination against external genital lesions was 79% and 94.4% against persistent infection.

- In 2009, the FDA approved the quadrivalent vaccine (Gardasil) for use in boys and men from 9 through 26 years to prevent prevention genital warts caused by HPV 6 and 11. However, the Advisory Committee on Immunization Practices (ACIP) holds this recommendation as a permissive utilization, meaning it is optional, and vaccination should be guided by a discussion between provider and patient, as opposed to a routine use of the vaccine.[32,33]

■ Future Questions

- ■ Duration of immunogenicity and clinical efficacy are unknown.
  - One study showed that, at 5 years after vaccination with the quadrivalent vaccine, stable anti-HPV levels were seen as well as a robust immune memory, suggesting that efficacy would be long-lasting.[17]
  - Seropositivity is not a good predictor of clinical efficacy. One study showed 40% of quadrivalent vaccinated women were anti-HPV 18 seronegative at the end of study although anti-HPV efficacy remained high (98.4%). The vaccine may induce protection via immune memory or lower-than-detectable antibody titers.[34]
- ■ The clinical effect of the vaccine on genital cancers has not been determined as the endpoints of the vaccine trials were preinvasive disease (CIN and adenocarcinoma in situ).
- ■ The clinical benefits for vaccinating women older than age 26 years are still unknown. The vaccine is believed to be immunogenic in an older population, but the cost effectiveness of vaccinating a lower risk population is unknown.
- ■ The quantity of antibodies needed for protection is unknown. Does a higher level translate to stronger

protection? There are no immune correlates to predict protection.

- Merck is currently testing an octavalent HPV vaccine.

- The current bivalent and quadrivalent vaccines do not provide a therapeutic effect for preexisting infection because infected basal cells do not express detectable levels of L1 or L2. It is estimated that it would take 20 years from the implementation of mass vaccination to see a change in cervical cancer rates worldwide. It will be important to develop a therapeutic vaccine as well because of the high prevalence of people infected with HPV 16 and 18.

- Studies are under way to investigate a two- versus three-dose vaccination, safety, and immunogenicity in HIV-positive people and efficacy in older women and in men.

■ References

1. Stanley M. Immunobiology of HPV and HPV vaccines. *Gynecol Oncol.* 2008;109(suppl):S15–S21.

2. Frazer IH, Cox JT, Mayeaux EJ Jr, et al. Advances in prevention of cervical cancer and other human papillomavirus-related diseases. *Pediatr Infect Dis J.* 2006;25(2)(suppl): S65–S81, quiz S82.

3. Schwarz TF, Leo O. Immune response to human papillomavirus after prophylactic vaccination with AS04-adjuvanted HPV-16/18 vaccine: improving upon nature. *Gynecol Oncol.* 2008;110(3)(suppl 1):S1–S10.

4. Eaton DK, Kann L, Kinchen S, et al. Youth risk behavior surveillance—United States, 2005. *MMWR Surveill Summ.* 2006;55:1–108.

5. Markowitz LE, Dunne EF, Saraiya M, et al. Quad-rivalent human papillomavirus vaccine: recommendations of the Advisory Committee on Immunization Practices (ACIP). *MMWR Recomm Rep.* 2007;56(RR-2):1–24.

6. Nardelli-Haefliger D, Wirthner D, Schiller JT, et al. Specific antibody levels at the cervix during the menstrual cycle of women vaccinated with human papillomavirus 16 virus-like particles. *J Natl Cancer Inst.* 2003;95:1128–1137.

7. Roberts JN, Buck CB, Thompson CD, et al. Genital transmission of HPV in a mouse model is potentiated by nonoxynol-9 and inhibited by carrageenan. *Nat Med.* 2007;13: 857–861.

8. Block SL, Nolan T, Sattler C, et al. Comparison of the immunogenicity and reactogenicity of a prophylactic quadrivalent

human papillomavirus (types 6, 11, 16, and 18) L1 virus-like particle vaccine in male and female adolescents and young adult women. *Pediatrics*. 2006;118:2135–2145.

9. Garland SM, Hernandez-Avila M, Wheeler CM. Quadrivalent vaccine against human papillomavirus to prevent anogenital diseases. *N Engl J Med*. 2007;356:1928–1943.

10. Paavonen J, Jenkins D, Bosch FX, et al. Efficacy of a prophylactic adjuvanted bivalent L1 virus-like-particle vaccine against infection with human papillomavirus types 16 and 18 in young women: an interim analysis of a phase III double-blind, randomised controlled trial. *Lancet*. 2007;369:2161–2170. [Erratum, *Lancet*. 2007;370:1414.].

11. Reisinger KS, Block SL, Lazcano-Ponce E, et al. Safety and persistent immunogenicity of a quadrivalent human papillomavirus types 6, 11, 16, 18 L1 virus-like particle vaccine in preadolescents and adolescents: a randomised controlled trial. *Pediatr Infect Dis J*. 2007;26:201–209.

12. The FUTURE II Study Group. Quadrivalent vaccine against human papilloma-virus to prevent high-grade cervical lesions. *N Engl J Med*. 2007;356:1915–1927.

13. Joura EA, Leodolter S, Hernandez-Avila M, et al. Efficacy of a quadrivalent prophylactic human papillomavirus (types 6, 11, 16, and 18) L1 virus-like-particle vaccine against high-grade vulvar and vaginal lesions: a combined analysis of three randomized clinical trials. *Lancet*. 2007;369:1693–1702.

14. Harper D, Gall S, Naud P, et al. Sustained immunogenicity and high efficacy against HPV-16/18 related cervical neoplasia: long-term follow up through 6.4 years in women vaccinated with Cervarix [abstract]. Presented at: 39th annual meeting of the Society of Gynecologic Oncologists; March 9–12, 2008; Tampa, FL.

15. Harper DM, Franco EL, Wheeler CM, et al. Sustained efficacy up to 4.5 years of a bivalent L1 virus-like particle vaccine against human papillomavirus types 16 and 18: follow-up from a randomised control trial. *Lancet*. 2006;367:1247–1255.

16. Paavonen J, Naud P, Salmerón J, et al; and HPV PATRICIA Study Group, Greenacre M. Efficacy of human papillomavirus (HPV)-16/18 AS04-adjuvanted vaccine against cervical infection and precancer caused by oncogenic HPV types (PATRICIA): final analysis of a double-blind, randomised study in young women. *Lancet*. 2009;374(9686):301–314.

17. Olsson SE, Villa LL, Costa RL, et al. Induction of immune memory following administration of a prophylactic quadrivalent human papillomavirus (HPV) types 6/11/16/18 L1 virus-like particle (VLP) vaccine. *Vaccine*. 2007;25:4931–4939.

18. Centers for Disease Control and Prevention. *HPV Vaccine Information for Young Women*. Atlanta, GA: Centers for Disease Control and Prevention. http://www.cdc.gov/std/hpv/STDFact-HPV-vaccine-young-women.htm#hpvvac4. Accessed January 2, 2010.

19. US Food and Drug Administration. *Product Approval Information: Human Papillomavirus Quadrivalent (Types 6, 11, 16, 18) Vaccine, Recombinant*. Silver Spring, MD: US Food and Drug Administration; 2008. http://www.fda.gov/cber/products/gardasil.htm. Accessed October 22, 2009.

20. Future II Study Group, et al. Prophylactic efficacy of a quadrivalent human papillomavirus (HPV) vaccine in women with virological evidence of HPV infection. *J Infect Dis*. 2007;196(10):1438–1446.

21. Einstein M, Baron M, Levin M, et al. Comparison of the immunogenicity and safety of Cervarix™ and Gardasil® human papillomavirus (HPV) cervical cancer vaccines in healthy women aged 18–45 years. *Human Vaccin*. 2009;5:10:705–719.

22. Pedersen C, Petaja T, Strauss G, et al. Immunization of early adolescent females with human papillomavirus type 16 and 18 L1 virus-like particle vaccine containing ASO4 adjuvant. *J Adolesc Health*. 2007;40:564–571.

23. Schiffman M, Kjaer SK. Chapter 2: natural history of anogenital human papillo- mavirus infection and neoplasia. *J Natl Cancer Inst Monogr*. 2003;31:14–19.

24. Grainge MJ, Seth R, Guo L, et al. Cervical human papillomavirus screening among older women. *Emerg Infect Dis*. 2005;11(11):1680–1685.

25. Castle PE, Schiffman M, Herrero R, et al. A prospective study of age trends in cervical human papillomavirus acquisition and persistence in Guanacaste, Costa Rica. *J Infect Dis*. 2005;191(11):1808–1816.

26. Schwarz TF, Spaczynski M, Schneider A, et al. Immunogenicity and tolerability of an HPV-16/18 AS04-adjuvanted prophylactic cervical cancer vaccine in women aged 15–55 years. *Vaccine*. 2009;27(4):581–587.

27. Muñoz N, Manalastas R Jr, Pitisuttithum P. Safety, immunogenicity, and efficacy of quadrivalent human papillomavirus (types 6, 11, 16, 18) recombinant vaccine in women aged 24–45 years: a randomised, double-blind trial. *Lancet*. 2009; 373:1949–1957.

28. Villa LL, Costa RL, Petta CA, et al. Prophylactic quadrivalent human papillo- mavirus (types 6, 11, 16, and 18) L1 virus-like particle vaccine in young women: a randomised double-blind placebo-controlled multicentre phase II efficacy trial. *Lancet Oncol*. 2005;6:271–278.

29. Slade BA, Leidel L, Vellozzi C, et al. Postlicensure safety surveillance for quadrivalent human papillomavirus recombinant vaccine. *JAMA*. 2009;302(7):750–757.

30. Giuliano AR, Palefsky JM. The efficacy of quadrivalent HPV (types 6/11/16/18) vaccine in reducing the incidence of HPV infection and HPV-related genital disease in young men [abstract]. Presented at: EUROGIN [European Research Organization on Genital Infection] International Multidisciplinary Conference; November 12–15, 2008; Nice, France.

31. Giuliano AR, Palefsky J; for the Male Quadrivalent HPV Vaccine Efficacy Trial Study Group. The efficacy of quadrivalent (types 6/11/16/18) vaccine against HPV-related genital disease and infection in young men [abstract O-01.07]. Twenty-Fifth International Papillomavirus Congress; May 8–14, 2009; Malmo, Sweden.

32. US Food and Drug Administration. FDA approves new indication for Gardasil to prevent genital warts in men and boys. http://www.fda.gov/NewsEvents/Newsroom/PressAnnouncements/ucm187003.htm. Accessed May 17, 2010.

33. Advisory Committee on Immunization Practices (ACIP) Vaccines for Children Program. Vaccines to prevent human papilloma virus. Resolution No. 010/09-1. Adopted and effective October 21, 2009. http://www.cdc.gov/vaccines/programs/vfc/downloads/resolution/0608.hpv.pdf. Accessed May 17, 2010

34. Joura EA, Kjaer SK, Wheeler CM, et al. HPV antibody levels and clinical efficacy following administration of a prophylactic quadrivalent HPV vaccine. *Vaccine*. 2008; 26(52):6844–6851.

Index

Note: Page numbers followed by *t* indicate tables.